Dealing With Grief and Loss

ROBERT GRIFFITH

GRIEF AND TRUTH PUBLISHING
1356 ... Suite 210
by processnature Publishing Program

GRACE AND TRUTH PUBLISHING
PO Box 338, Gunnedah NSW 2380 Australia
www.graceandtruthpublishing.com.au

ISBN 978-0-6486439-3-7

Introduction

Grief and loss are universal experiences that touch the lives of every individual at some point. Whether it's the death of a loved one, the end of a very close relationship or the loss of a job, these are painful moments which can leave us overwhelmed, lost, and in need of comfort. In times of grief, many turn to their faith for solace and support.

For Christians, our belief in a compassionate and loving God provides a unique framework for us to understand and navigate the many complexities of grief. The Christian faith and the presence of God provide a source of comfort, hope and healing that guides us through the darkest times of our lives.

This is much more than just a phycological support system, our God is real and present at such times in a way which cannot compare to even the best support that the world can offer us.

In this booklet, we will explore the various aspects of Christian comfort for those experiencing grief and loss. We will also explore the stages of grief, some common reactions to loss, and stress the importance of allowing people to grieve.

We will also examine the biblical perspective on grief and loss; exploring the presence of God in times of sorrow; letting the Scriptures offer hope and comfort; and the role of prayer and faith in the healing process.

I will also provide some practical ways in which Christians can extend comfort to those who may be grieving. From active listening and empathy to providing emotional support and helping them with practical needs, we will discover how we can learn to be a source of comfort and strength to others.

By exploring these topics, I hope to provide at least some insight and guidance for Christians who wish to offer solace to those experiencing grief and loss.

Through a combination of some biblical wisdom and practical advice, we become an instrument of God's love and compassion in a world that often feels broken and hurting.

Understanding Grief and Loss

Grief is a complex and deeply personal experience that people encounter whenever they suffer some significant loss in their lives.

Whether it be the death of a loved one, the end of a relationship, or any other form of loss, grief is a natural response to these life-altering events.

In order to provide effective comfort and support to those experiencing grief, it is essential to have a basic understanding of the grieving process.

The Five Stages of Grief

The five stages of grief is a construct proposed by Elisabeth Kübler-Ross in her 1969 book, *On Death and Dying*. Since the release of the book, the five stages of grief have made their way into popular culture and people have gravitated towards the intuitive nature of the stages.

Here's an overview of the five stages and what each one represents.

Stage 1: Denial

This first stage can initially help you survive the loss. It's kind of like a built-in defence mechanism.

In this initial stage you might think life makes no sense, has no real meaning, and is just too overwhelming. You start to deny the reality of what has happened and, in effect, go numb.

It's common in this stage to wonder how life will go on after this loss. You are in a state of shock; life as you knew it has changed completely in an instant, and sometimes without any warning.

If you were diagnosed with a deadly disease, you might believe the news is not correct - maybe a mistake has occurred somewhere in the lab - they mixed up your blood work with someone else. If you receive news of the death of a loved one, you perhap will cling to a false hope that they identified the wrong person. This is a natural gut response, "Surely, this cannot be true!"

In the denial stage, you are not living in reality, you you are living in a 'prefered' reality. Interestingly, it is denial and shock that help you survive and cope with the grief event in these early days. Denial aids in pacing your feelings of grief. Instead of becoming overwhelmed with grief, we deny it and stagger its full impact on us at one time.

Think of it as your body's natural defences saying "hey, there's only so much I can handle at once." Once the denial and shock begin to fade, the real healing process can begin. At this point, those feelings that you were once suppressing will start coming to the surface.

Stage 2: Anger

Once you start to live in reality again and not in a fantasy, anger might set in. This is a common time to think "why me?" and "life's not fair!"

You might want to blame others for the cause of your grief and also may redirect your anger to close friends and family.

You find it incomprehensible that something like this could happen to you. If you are strong in your faith, you might start to question your belief in God. *"Where is God? Why didn't He protect me?"*

Researchers and mental health experts agree that anger is a very difficult, but really necessary stage of the grieving process.

Encourage the anger. It's important to truly feel the anger. Even though it might seem like you are in an endless cycle of anger, it will dissipate - and the more you truly feel the anger, the more quickly it will dissipate, and the more quickly you will heal. It's very uncomfortable for you and even more so sometimes for those close to you, who may bear the brunt of your anger, but it has a purpose and it is not healthy to suppress your feelings of anger.

Anger is a natural response and arguably, a very necessary one. When you experience a grief event, you might feel disconnected from reality, as if you have no grounding anymore.

Your life has shattered and there's nothing solid to hold on to. Think of anger as a strength to bind you to reality. You might feel deserted or abandoned during a grief event - that no one casres are you're alone in this world. That's usually not true, but it is how you feel at this stage of the grieving process.

The releasing of that anger is what might provide a bridge back to reality for you and connect you to people again. As hard as it is to experience or see in others, it is a natural step in healing – provided it does not last too long.

Stage 3: Bargaining

When something terrible happens, have you ever caught yourself making a deal with God? "Please God, if you heal my husband, I will strive to be the best wife I can ever be – and never complain again." It can take many forms.

This is bargaining. In a way, this stage is a waste of energy and provides nothing but false hope.

You might fool yourself into believing that you can avoid the grief through a type of negotiation with God. "If you change this, I'll change that." You are desperate to get your life back to how it was before the grief event, so you are willing to make a major life change in an attempt to regain normality.

Guilt is a common wingman of bargaining. This is when you may endure the endless instances of "If only .." *"If only I had left the house just a minute sooner the accident would have never happened. If only I had encouraged him to go to the doctor six months ago like I first thought, the cancer could have been found sooner and he could have been saved."* This stage can be very damaging if we stay there too long – but it's inevitable for many people.

Stage 4: Depression

Depression is a commonly accepted form of grief. Most people associate depression immediately with grief - as it is a 'present' emotion. It represents the emptiness we feel when we are living in reality and realize that the person or situation is gone or come to an end. In this stage, you might withdraw from life, feel numb, live in a fog, and not even want to get out of bed each day.

The world might seem overwhelming or too much for you to face. You don't want to be around others; don't feel like talking; and experience feelings of hopelessness. You might even experience suicidal thoughts - thinking "what's the point of going on?"

Again, this stage may not be avoidable, however, it is perhaps the most serious stage in that some people get trapped here and don't move past it and reach acceptance. This is when professional help may need to be secured to help you or the person you are supporting in grief to gain the tools they need to conquer the depression.

Stage 5: Acceptance

The last stage of grief identified by Kübler-Ross is acceptance. Not in the sense that "it's okay my husband died" but rather, "my husband died, but I am going to be okay." In this stage, your emotions may begin to stabilize as you re-enter reality.

You come to terms with the fact that in this 'new' reality, your partner is never coming back or that you are going to succumb to your illness and die soon - and you're okay with that now. You accept the reality which has been given to you.

This is not a 'good' thing - but it's something you will learn to live with and embrace. It may involve a long time of adjustment. There will be good days, there will be bad days, and then there will be good days again. In this stage, it does not mean you'll never have another bad day where you are feel so uncontrollably sad. But the good days will start to outnumber the bad days - it does gets better.

In this stage, you finally emerge from your fog; you start to engage with friends again; and you might even make new relationships as time goes on. You finally accept and understand that your loved one can never be replaced, but you move, grow, and evolve into your new reality.

Grief is a very complex experience that is walked through independently by each person who finds themselves on this path. The five stages of grief created by Ross are a representation of the most common emotions and experiences faced and traversed by people she encountered while she was working with terminally ill patients.

The stages have been criticized because of their linear progression where one stage leads into the next. But they are not meant to be seen this way.

We know that the stages are fluid and that people experience many of the stages at different times or simultaneously. The order in which people move in and out of the stages is based on the individual and is not mapped out with precise certainty. There is no formula for the time a person spends in each stage. We are all different and we will all respond to grief differently. Some people don't experience some of these stages at all and still recover.

The stages of grief simply give us an umbrella view of the different emotions and behaviours that we might expect when encountering a serious loss. Grief is commonly misunderstood or misplaced by the person experiencing it as depression.

In my many years in pastoral ministry, I have often sat with people who are explaining their symptoms of depression dealing with grief and don't know it. This is no fault of the person, we just assume that depression is a stand-alone mental health issue when, more often than not, it is really the outcome of something else that is happening to us or in us.

Without doubt, loss and grief are a primary trigger for depression and until we properly deal with the grief, the depression will never leave us.

Common Reactions to Loss

In addition to the stages of grief, there are common reactions and emotions that we may experience when faced with loss. These reactions often vary greatly from person to person, but here are four of the most common ones:

Intense sadness ...

Grief often brings about deep sadness and this profound sense of loss. This sadness can at times be overwhelming and might manifest in physical symptoms such as difficulty sleeping, fatigue, and a loss of appetite. Recognising these issues as the effects of grief can help us better deal with them.

Anguish and yearning ...

Individuals may experience a strong desire to be reunited with the person or reality they have lost. This yearning can be accompanied by feelings of intense longing and aching.

It makes no sense because they know that ship has sailed and there is no going back ... but the feelings are still real. It's the emotional equivalent of 'phantom limb' pain.

Guilt and self-blame ...

It is not uncommon for individuals to feel guilt or self-blame after a loss. They may question their actions or decisions leading up to the loss, even if they were not directly responsible. This can be very debilitating and a person should not remain in this place too long – it can be destructive. They may even need professional help.

Anxiety and fear ...

The experience of loss can often shake a person's sense of security and control, leading to increased levels of anxiety and fear about the future. They may worry about additional losses or struggle with feelings of vulnerability. This is perfectly normal and usually will pass with the passage of time.

The Importance of Grieving

While grief can be very painful, it's an essential and natural part of the healing process. It is important to allow individuals to grieve and not rush them through the process. We should allow people to acknowledge and process their emotions, adjust to the changed reality, and ultimately find a way to move forward.

They can't do that while their well-meaning family or friends are trying to help them 'move on' and 'get over it.' The process of grief should certainly not go on forever, but it should never be rushed either.

Biblical Perspective on Grief and Loss

Grief and loss are universal experiences that touch the lives of every human being at some point. The Christian faith offers a unique support in these very challenging times, providing comfort, hope, and guidance through the lens of the Bible.

The most reassuring aspect of the Christian faith is our belief in God's presence during times of grief. The Bible assures us that God is always close to the broken-hearted and those mourn.

Even in our darkest moments, we can find solace in knowing that God is with us, providing His loving support and understanding. God's presence is the only thing which can bring most of us through grief, stronger, wiser and with greater faith.

If we are not able to discern the presence of God with us at our time of greatest need, the journey through grief can be a truly treacherous one.

The Bible is filled with verses that offer comfort and hope to those who are experiencing grief and loss. These Scriptures can serve as a source of strength and encouragement during difficult times.

Passages like Psalm 23, which speaks of God as a shepherd Who guides and comforts us, or Isaiah 41:10, which reassures us of God's presence and strength, can bring immense solace to those who are hurting.

Additionally, the New Testament presents Jesus as someone Who experienced grief Himself. In the book of John, we read about the death of Lazarus, and how Jesus wept for his friend (John 11:35). This shows that Jesus understands our pain and sorrow, and through His example, we find a great reassurance that we are never alone in our grief.

The Role of Prayer and Faith

There is no doubt that prayer and faith both play essential roles in navigating grief and loss from a Christian perspective. Through prayer we are able to communicate with God, pouring out our fears and emotions. It's a way to find solace in God's presence and seek His guidance and comfort.

Having faith means trusting in God's plan and His ability to bring healing and restoration. It requires us to believe that even in the midst of our pain, God is working for our good (Romans 8:28). Our faith will provide a foundation of hope which enables us to persevere through the grieving process, knowing that there is light at the end of the tunnel.

By embracing the biblical perspective on grief and loss, Christians can find great strength, comfort and hope in the midst of their pain. The assurance of God's presence, the wisdom of Scripture, and the power of prayer and faith all combine to offer a solid foundation for navigating the very challenging journey through grief.

Practical Ways to Comfort Those in Grief

One of the most important ways to comfort those who are grieving is through active listening and a genuine empathy. When someone is grieving, they may need a safe space to express their emotions and share their memories.

As a Christian, it is essential to provide a listening ear without judgment or interruption and always resisting the temptation to give advice.

Allow the grieving person to talk about their loss, their emotions and their experiences without the feeling of being rushed or dismissed.

Active listening involves giving your full attention to the person speaking. Maintain eye contact, nod in understanding, and provide verbal cues to show that you are present and engaged with them. Try to avoid distractions, such as checking your phone or thinking about what you will say next.

Remember, this moment is all about the person who is grieving, and your role is to offer comfort and support – not pat answers or advice.

Empathy is the ability to understand and share the feelings of another person, putting yourself in their shoes and trying to imagine the depth of their pain. You can express empathy by simply saying, "I can't imagine how difficult this must be for you," or "I am here for you, and I want to support you in any way I can." You need to acknowledge their pain and let them know that their emotions are valid.

In addition to active listening and empathy, being able to provide emotional support is crucial when comforting someone in going through grief.

This may involve offering a shoulder to cry on, and being present during their moments of sadness, or simply being available whenever they need to talk or vent. Grief can be isolating, and having someone who is willing to be there unconditionally can make a significant difference in their healing process.

It's important to understand that everyone grieves differently. Some people may find solace in talking about their loss, while others may prefer silence or distraction. Be sensitive to their needs and respect their boundaries. Let them know that you will be available to listen or provide support, but also make sure you allow them the space to grieve in their own way and at their own pace.

When someone is grieving, everyday tasks can at times become overwhelming and burdensome. As a Christian seeking to comfort those in grief, you could offer some practical assistance which can be a tremendous help at such times.

This could include tasks such as preparing meals, running errands, or taking care of some household chores. By helping this way you can alleviate some of the stress and allow the grieving person the time and space to focus on their healing.

Additionally, you can offer to accompany them to appointments, assist with funeral arrangements, or help with paperwork if needed. By providing this practical support, you are demonstrating your love and care in a tangible way, making a difficult time a little more manageable for the person in grief.

Remember, it is essential to ask before taking any action. Don't overstep the mark. Some individuals may prefer to handle practical tasks themselves, while others may welcome the assistance.

You should respect their choices and let them guide you in determining how you can best support them in their time of need.

In conclusion, comforting those experiencing grief and loss requires a very compassionate approach, grounded in active listening, emotional support, empathy and practical assistance. As Christians, we are called to embody Christ's love and to be a source of comfort to those in need.

By understanding the stages of grief, embracing a biblical perspective, and employing practical ways to comfort, we can help individuals navigate their grief journey and find solace and healing in the midst of their pain.

Let us now extend that comfort to those who are grieving and offer them the healing touch of God's love. In doing so, we can bring light into the darkest corners of their life and provide a glimpse of hope to those who really need it most.

- - - - - - - - - - - - - - - -

"Praise be to the God and Father of our Lord Jesus Christ, the Father of compassion and the God of all comfort, who comforts us in all our troubles, so that we can comfort those in any trouble with the comfort we ourselves receive from God. For just as we share abundantly in the sufferings of Christ, so also our comfort abounds through Christ."

2 Corinthians 1:3-5 (NIV)

www.ingramcontent.com/pod-product-compliance
Lightning Source LLC
Chambersburg PA
CBHW072102040426
42334CB00041B/2061